RAYMOND RANDOLPH

CHIROPRACTOR

The Essential Guide to Chiropractic Care, Learn All About
the Science Behind Chiropractic Care and Its Benefits in
Pain Relief and Improved Immune System

Descrierea CIP a Bibliotecii Naţionale a României
RAYMOND RANDOLPH
CHIROPRACTOR. The Essential Guide to Chiropractic
Care, Learn All About the Science Behind Chiropractic Care
and Its Benefits in Pain Relief and Improved Immune System /
Raymond Randolph – Bucharest: Editura My Ebook, 2020
    ISBN

RAYMOND RANDOLPH

CHIROPRACTOR

The Essential Guide to Chiropractic Care, Learn All About the Science Behind Chiropractic Care and Its Benefits in Pain Relief and Improved Immune System

My Ebook Publishing House
Bucharest, 2020

TABLE OF CONTENTS

INTRODUCTION

Chiropractic care is more than you think. You probably are well aware of the popularized image that chiropractic care has in the media. It has to do with the dramatic popping of joints and the awkward positioning of the body while this is taking place. You know of the ample pressure applied to the patient to help improve a bad back, but there is more.

Did you know that chiropractic care is for more than just back pain and neck pain? Did you know that chiropractic care can help your headaches? Did you know that chiropractic care may be able to improve conditions that are beyond the scope of musculature issues and may even be able to improve your overall health?

Its history begins at least as far back as recorded history with the healers of those times aware of a connection between the health of the spine and the health of the individual. It continues into the modern world where chiropractors are put through extensive training to be licensed to diagnose and treat problems within the body.

The benefits of chiropractic care may not even now be fully known. The benefits begin with the management of pain and go from there. They include an improvement of the functioning of your immune system as well as a laundry list of other benefits that are directly linked to your overall well being.

The science of chiropractic care is growing as the field receives increased attention. Once relegated to treating primarily back and neck pain, now this field is developing into an instrument to promote overall health.

While still effective in treating the often serious conditions of back and neck pain, there may be much more that this alternative method of healing can accomplish.

Chiropractic philosophy does not see problems within the body as isolated events. It sees the body as one integrated, cohesive whole where a symptom in one part of the body suggests that a closer look at the entire system is an advantageous and perhaps even a necessary next step.

The field of chiropractic care continues to gain support both in the form of popularity and in the form of research. As the field of health care continues to look for alternative forms of healing the body and helping the body to heal itself, chiropractic care will continue to be an area of study that will be explored because of its understanding of the integrated nature of the human body and its ability to work with that integrated nature to promote healing.

1

A BACKGROUND OF CHIROPRACTIC CARE

The world's understanding of the implications of chiropractic care is still in its early stages even though knowledge of chiropractic science has been around to some degree as long as recorded time. While many civilizations throughout time have understood and recognized that on some level the health and positioning of the spine is related to the health of the individual, the modern world is only now beginning to gain a more complete understanding of what this might mean.

Today, chiropractic science is often thought of as a way to improve back problems and other such examples of physical pain, but this is only the start. Chiropractic science extends beyond problems of pain as related to musculoskeletal issues into the very realm of overall human health. From pain relief to immunity and general well being, chiropractic care is at the core of health knowledge.

No discussion of health, both maintenance and recovery, is complete without a mention of the health of this pivotal bodily system. The spine exerts its influence into all parts of the body as an integrated whole and consequently is a main figure in maintaining and achieving a healthy state. The repercussions of the health of the spine as they relate to overall health are beginning to be introduced into the collective consciousness, but these ideas are far from new.

A HISTORY OF CHIROPRACTIC CARE

The history of chiropractic care extends at least as far back as written records exist. Writings that found their birthplaces in China and Greece spoke of chiropractic techniques wherein adjustment of the spine was used to ameliorate back pain.

The famous Greek physician Hippocrates even weighed in on the topic of chiropractic care. He once wrote, "Get knowledge of the spine for that is the requisite for many diseases." Even he saw the connection between the health of the spine, spinal manipulation, and overall health. This connection has been identified since the start of recorded time.

It was not until the later part of the nineteenth century that the theories and practices of chiropractic care started to be fully acknowledged in the United States. As the twentieth century began and progressed, chiropractic care grew as a recognized and respected part of the health care field. There have been numerous studies inquiring into the efficacy of this type of medical care with pleasing results.

This is excellent news considering the prevalence of conditions that can benefit from chiropractic care. Back pain issues rank as the second most common cause of individuals visiting their doctors. It also ranks highly on the list of reasons why individuals miss work. In fact, approximately half of working Americans have stated that they experience some form of back pain. Given these statistics, the burgeoning interest in chiropractic care seems to be fortuitously timed.

This leads one to wonder what causes these widespread problems that find their source in the spine. More than that, it leads to a contemplation of how these problems may be treated or even prevented. Knowledge of chiropractic care leads not only to chiropractic treatment itself but also to an awareness of the importance of spinal alignment and how individuals may take better care of themselves so that pain and problems caused by spinal misalignment may be averted.

It is said that a great deal of this growing popularity is owed to the non- invasive nature of chiropractic techniques. It is thought to be a natural, healthy alternative in some cases to the more invasive methods often favored in Western medicine. Chiropractic care is not only though to help heal individuals but to help their bodies heal themselves. This, in itself, is revolutionary.

With all the advances in medical technology, one has to wonder if there is any technology so impressive, so intricate, and so effective as that present in the human body. Its innate knowledge and ability to heal itself is not yet completely understood, and any practice that can allow the body's ability to heal to be fully realized has almost limitless potential.

Chiropractic care seeks to assist the body's natural healing potential, and does so in a non-invasive manner. The implications of such treatment are extensive. What better way to work towards healing than to help a body help itself?

EDUCATIONAL REQUIREMENTS FOR CHIROPRACTORS

The required education for chiropractors consists of four to five years at a chiropractic college with the appropriate accreditation. This course of study includes at least 4,200 hours of experience in the classroom, in the laboratory, and in direct clinical activity. About 555 of these hours are dedicated to having students learn about observing and analyzing the spine as well as on the actual spinal adjustments that are so characteristic of this field.

Although the curriculum for chiropractors is heavily focused on exclusively chiropractic concerns, it also includes a delving into clinical sciences and general health topics. This serves to educate students in a deeper understanding of the human body as a whole and how disease functions as a malfunction in the body.

The integrated nature of the human body makes this training essential. With the far reaching implications of chiropractic care and its spinal adjustments, a thorough understanding of the mechanisms of both illness and health is necessary for those who wish to practice. This explains why their curriculum includes courses such as physiology and biochemistry as well as differential diagnoses and radiology.

A well-rounded education assures that the doctor holds a comprehensive understanding of the body's natural function and the ways in which disease interferes with that functioning. The nature of chiropractic care necessitates this all encompassing curriculum. To treat health problems effectively, one must first understand what one is dealing with.

In addition to treating musculoskeletal issues, chiropractors may provide information regarding rehabilitation to patients such as exercises to help recovery along. They are also able to provide information in areas such as nutrition. This is especially pertinent if weight is affecting the curvature of the spine. Knowing that health is a result of a complete lifestyle and not isolated factors, chiropractors learn to look at the big picture.

Even all this training is not the end of the student's journey. Chiropractic students must then pass the national exam, any local exams, and meet the licensing requirements that may be required by the state or states where they intend to practice. As a result of this training and licensing, chiropractors have the ability to not only treat but also to diagnose patients as they are doctors.

The extensive training is understandable and necessary when one considers the relative fragility of the spinal cord when it is being directly manipulated in this way. The rigorous course of study designed for chiropractors ensures that their understanding is sufficient to allow them to heal without harming the patient. Rearranging the positioning of the spinal column requires a depth of knowledge that can only be obtained by such an intense curriculum. This cursory explanation fails to capture the truly rigorous nature of chiropractic study but gives a small window into a world where students learn to manipulate the spine and, with it, the health of the entire body. They learn to quite literally hold a patient's health in their hands.

2

WHAT IS CHIROPRACTIC CARE?

What is chiropractic care? Is it effective? Who can benefit from chiropractic care? All these questions are at the forefront of a patient's mind when he or she considers chiropractic treatment as an option. While it may be a less traditional mode of treating conditions than medication and surgery, chiropractic care certainly deserves a second look.

Chiropractic care is often thought of as an alternative route of treating injuries involving the spine and the surrounding musculature. Its applications may not be limited to affecting these particular health issues, but these are the most common applications.

Injuries involving the spine and the surrounding musculature can often be treated with a combination of

17

medications and surgery, but is this the only way to deal with such injuries? Is chiropractic care a viable option for those who wish to pursue a non-invasive treatment modality? The answer to these questions begins with a look at the purpose and practice of chiropractic care.

Chiropractic care is often only a part of an all inclusive treatment regimen. A chiropractor begins by taking a patient's health history, performing an examination, running the necessary tests, and evaluating a patient. It is from this point that the chiropractor proceeds to make a diagnosis, if appropriate, and to decide the best course of treatment for a patient.

Through an accurate diagnosis and the proper follow up, a chiropractor seeks to ameliorate or even repair conditions that involve the spine. What constitutes a condition involving the spine may not have reached a consensus in the medical community as of yet, but the fact that the spinal column serves a function in various systems throughout the body as a gateway or messenger service, if you will, leads medical professionals and lay people alike to wonder where the health of the spine ends and the health of the body as a complete entity begins.

The spinal manipulation itself is the method through which the chiropractor seeks to realign and return the spine to its natural healthy structure. This is the well known application of pressure to the body to reorganize and realign the spinal structure. This structure, when returned to its proper alignment, allows the body to carry out all of its tasks more effectively.

This process may be accomplished in a single visit although it often takes repeat visits that may last for weeks or even years. The patient is often seen on a weekly basis for treatments in an effort to retrain the spine to assume proper positioning within the body.

The duration and frequency of treatment is decided on a case by case basis and all depends upon the needs of the patient. It also depends upon the reason for the treatment. The treatment may be administered for an acute condition, for a chronic or ongoing condition, or as a preventative measures. Any overview given has to begin with the knowledge that no two patients are completely alike and will not necessarily require the same course of treatment.

The reason why a person may seek out or be seen by a chiropractor is usually for pain management or resolution. It may also be for reasons regarding an individual's range of motion. People tend to seek out medical care when there are outward signs of a condition within the body, and pain is at the forefront of reasons to seek out chiropractic care. It is also pain issues with the musculature of the body that are primarily associated with chiropractic treatment so it stands to reason that this would be the main reason to find such care.

These injuries may be the result of repetitive stress injuries, a pinched nerve, an acute trauma, or any of a long list of other possible causes. Whatever the reason, the interior problem has developed to the extent where it is now presenting with exterior symptoms that cannot be ignored. At this point, the patient is forced to seek some form of treatment to avoid the unpleasant and possibly painful symptoms.

Basically, the process of treatment begins when a patient has a problem, usually pain, and is seeking relief. That is where the chiropractor comes in, but what are the mechanisms by which this process works?

THE SCIENCE BEHIND CHIROPRACTIC CARE

Everyone has that image from television, movies, and possibly real chiropractic experiences of a chiropractor cracking a patient's back, but what does this really do? How does correcting the positioning of the spine affect the body in any appreciable way? To grasp the purpose of spinal realignment, you must first understand the basic way in which the body works and how the brain and the rest of the body are connected.

Think of the basic science of the body. The brain is the start of it all. The brain sends out a signal every time a part of the body needs to do anything. If you want to lift your arm then the brain sends a signal down to your arm to tell it to move. If there is food in your stomach then the brain send a signal to tell your stomach to produce digestive juices. If your brain is going to know what is going on in the body so that it can send out the appropriate signals then it has to be able to receive signals back from the body as well.

This is clearly an oversimplified explanation but more than adequate to illustrate the following point. The brain

21

sends signals for the production of neurotransmitters, the operation of various organs, the secretion of digestive juices, and everything else that goes on in the body basically, but how do these messages get where they are going?

They are sent through the spinal cord. The spinal cord is the route that these messages take to make their way to various parts of the body so that they can be received and carried out. A spine that is in perfect health and that is perfectly aligned allows for an unobstructed pathway through which these signals from the brain can be transmitted.

If, however, the spine is not in proper alignment then these signals cannot travel as efficiently or even as effectively to their chosen destinations.

Orders sent from the brain may not be carried out as quickly or as effectively. In severe cases, they may not be carried out at all.

Usually, these messages seem to be transmitted instantaneously. You do not need to think about wanting to move your arm and then wait for the signal to travel. It happens so quickly that you lift your arm with barely a thought and without hesitation.

The messages sent from the brain travel so quickly that you do not think about how a signal gets from your brain to another part of your body. It just does. The slowing of the signals sent from the brain is a common and inevitable occurrence with spinal misalignment. This means that every part of the body that receives signals from or sends signals to the brain will be adversely affected. That basically means every part of the body.

When considering this, you can understand how a misaligned spine could lead to problems in various parts of the body. Because the messages that are sent through the spinal cord make their way to all parts of the body, a multitude of problems in the body could find their causation, totally or partially, within the spinal cord itself.

The realignment of the spinal cord, such as that done through chiropractic care, could serve to ameliorate or to reverse any conditions caused by this misalignment. A pain in one part of the body may seem to be located solely in that part, but the affliction may actually find its cause in the spinal cord. If the cause does indeed exist in the spinal cord then any other treatment that ignores this causation could prove to be ineffective or may merely serve as a way to mask symptoms while allowing the true cause to go untreated.

The specifics of this process may be best left to the professionals, but this general overview allows you to imagine the extent to which the alignment of your spine may be affecting your health.

Even if the spine is not causing a particular condition then the natural action that your body would take to heal itself could be impeded by problems with or misalignment of your spine. The body's ability to heal depends upon these signals because that is another action that is carried out by the body, albeit an often invisible one.

When the body is without its natural healing capabilities, problems are bound to manifest, and conditions seem destined to deteriorate. To put it simply, spinal misalignment places pressure on the nerves, disrupting signals and keeping the body from working and healing as it should.

On the other hand, a properly aligned spine sends signals quickly and easily. The body functions at peak efficiency, and no problems result from poor spinal positioning. The body can perform its duties, both seen and unseen, and can exercise its remarkable capacity to heal itself. The importance of this clear communication and the resultant proper functioning of the body cannot be overestimated.

The implications of this knowledge are far reaching. The domino effect that could find its beginning in the spine makes this an important aspect of health care. A misaligned spine could be creating problems in the body, and it may be preventing the body from effectively healing itself.

This would indicate that the need for outside measures could be created, and possibly eliminated, by a resolution of these precipitating factors. The very cause of a problem may also be inhibiting the recovery from that problem. By taking care of the cause, you may be speeding up recovery and preventing not only that problem but future problems as well.

On the other hand, if signals sent from the brain are not received or are not received as efficiently as they should be then the body cannot hope to operate at its best. This leaves the body in a more vulnerable state and increases the chances that minor conditions will become major and that major conditions will require extensive intervention from outside of the body.

Without its unencumbered capacity to protect itself, the body becomes predisposed towards all manner of unfortunate conditions. More than that, without its ability to heal itself, those unfortunate conditions become threats that the body is ill-equipped to deal with. The body can progress to a state where it is just short ofbeing defenseless.

The lesson that can be learned from this is that the health of the spine can serve as an indication of the health of the entire body. Chiropractic care takes this knowledge and works toward a resolution of not only immediate issues but also toward a restoration of overall proper spinal alignment.

The next logical question is how this is accomplished.

3

WHAT DO CHIROPRACTORS DO EXACTLY?

First and foremost, chiropractors evaluate an individual. They seek to diagnose any possible problems and, of course, seek out causes for the problem that brought the patient in. This evaluation begins with a thorough health history for the patient and then continues with a complete physical evaluation, possibly including x-rays for a more complete picture of any abnormalities. Then the chiropractor continues based on the information gathered. Assuming that this step has been completed and it has been ascertained that the patient will benefit from chiropractic care then the real work begins.

Chiropractors crack backs. This is not all there is to it, but it is a good starting point. Chiropractors actually perform spinal manipulation on patients. This manipulation seeks to restore the proper alignment of the spine and, with it, the patient's health. By health, this primarily means an improvement in the condition that caused the patient to seek treatment in the first place although this act of spinal manipulation can be used as a preventative measure and a way to improve overall health.

It is good to mention now that if a chiropractor does not feel that chiropractic treatment is the appropriate method of treatment then the chiropractor will refer the patient to an expert in another, more appropriate field. Chiropractic care can be helpful in many instances but not necessarily all. When chiropractic care is not the method of choice then the patient will be referred to another specialist. Chiropractic care is often used in conjunction with other forms of treatment.

If chiropractic care is the appropriate method of treatment then the chiropractor uses techniques of spinal manipulation. The process of restoring proper spinal alignment may seem rather simple and even a bit simplistic, but the effects are far reaching.

The process of spinal realignment is sought out through adjustments. During an adjustment, a chiropractor applies sufficient pressure to joints to give them back their mobility and to give them a chance to properly heal. This application of pressure is the common method of affecting changes in spinal alignment.

What chiropractors do is try to seek out the root cause of the symptoms that a patient experiencing. They do not content themselves with the simplest method of pain management, such as medication, although other avenues including medication may be used as adjuncts to chiropractic treatment. Instead, they seek the problem at its source so that the weed may be pulled out at the root and balance may be restored. The restoration of balance is the key. Medication may be used to help manage symptoms, but it is viewed as a temporary measure. The end goal is to correct the problem so that the patient may function without medicinal aid. Every case is different so this may not always be possible or advisable.

The chiropractor does not just look for the source of the immediate problems, however. They will also make an appraisal of the spine as a whole to discover any and all problems that could benefit from chiropractic care. Today's spinal misalignment could lead to tomorrow's health issues. By catching them early, these problems of tomorrow have a chance to be corrected before they become fully realized.

Pain may be averted and treatment is often simpler in all fields of medicine when problems are caught early.

Ideally, the action of spinal manipulation will serve on an immediate level to restore mobility to joints. When they have reached a state of restricted range of motion, joints may produce discomfort. Restoring the range of motion and releasing the tension that builds up from pain and disuse can provide relief. On a larger level, this process of spinal manipulation will also hopefully allow the damage to heal even as pain is lessened and mobility is restored.

This damage or pain may be the result of a tissue injury. This tissue injury may have been caused by a single event, an acute trauma, or it may be the result of repetitive actions that have stressed the body. This precipitating situation may have included a person remaining in a stationary position with poor posture for extended periods of time or some form of awkward repetitive hand movements that were also paired with poor posture.

The result of such an injury is pain and inflammation along with an often decreased range of motion in the affected joints. The purpose of chiropractic care is returning these joints to their natural state of functioning, restoring range of motion, decreasing pain, and permitting the affected tissues to heal.

THE TRUTH ABOUT ADJUSTMENTS

You might wonder if a patient will feel pain while these adjustments are being performed. The majority of patients will not. There may be some slight discomfort initially as they adjust to the treatment process, but this is minor and will pass. Actually, many patients report a rapid sensation of relief following adjustments for the conditions that they seek treatment for.

As stated earlier, the chiropractor does not merely seek to treat the condition that a patient came in for but checks for any misalignments that may be present. This way any possible problems or positioning that could lead to future problems are all treated. The treatment is not limited to attempts at treating the problem at hand.

In fact, it is not uncommon for patients to experience an improvement in symptoms that they thought were unrelated to their original complaint or just in their overall feeling of well being. The integrated nature of the body and the way that the spine influences the body as a whole makes this a very real occurrence.

Adjustments may be used be used to deal with acute conditions, chronic conditions, or they may be used as more of a preventative measure. A patient does not necessarily need to wait until a problem is fully developed before seeking out treatment for spinal misalignment.

Developing or potential conditions may be caught early and rectified before they can come to fruition. Also, the general health and feeling of well being may be improved through chiropractic intervention even if there is not one discernable problem to treat. Because of the all inclusive nature of spinal health, preventative chiropractic adjustments are thought to be quite beneficial for many patients.

During the course of a session, the chiropractor introduces the appropriate amount of pressure using their hands to the patient's body to complete each adjustment. This is where the extensive curriculum that a chiropractor undergoes when training pays off. These somewhat simple movements require a comprehensive background in physiology and related subjects to be performed correctly and safely.

A patient may find it disconcerting to hear a loud cracking or popping noise coming from joints as adjustments are made. This sound is created by small amounts of gas being moved about the joints during the adjustments. The movement of the gas creates the sound. This sound may not always be present when an adjustment is made and is not an indication of the efficacy of the treatment.

It is similar to a person cracking their knuckles. The release of the gas creates the cracking sound and does not necessarily indicate anything more that the movement of the gas.

The amount of force required to complete an adjustment is not the same from one patient to the next. The amount of pressure necessary to perform the appropriate spinal adjustment depends largely on the person and the adjustment to be made.

If the problems are concentrated in the neck then a chiropractor may focus efforts in that area. Cervical adjustments are utilized to free up the neck muscles, relieving the tension that may be present and aiding the mobility of the neck. Clearly, neck adjustments are not likely to require as much force as adjustments performed on the lower parts of the spine. It is the chiropractor's training that allows for the assessment of the situation and the application of the correct amount of force.

Although the popularized image of chiropractic care may be one that includes a loud cracking or popping sound, the force applied varies and is highly controlled. The amount of force necessary to create changes in one person may be too much for another and what is the right amount of force for another person may not be sufficient for yet another. The treatment, while consistent, is individualized.

Chiropractors require the physical strength to make the necessary adjustments. The amount of strength needed may vary depending on the individual patient and the adjustments that are necessary. The physicality of this profession is another prerequisite for chiropractors. They have to not only know how to perform the adjustments but be physically able to complete them as well.

These actions are not intended to cause the patient any pain although they may result in a feeling of soreness for a patient. This soreness is often likened to the feeling a person has after an exercise session.

Some patients may wonder if they are able to perform adjustments on themselves. Often individuals can create a similar popping sound with their joints if they try. This is not advisable. Chiropractic adjustments are precise and require years of study to perform correctly. The creation of this popping or cracking sound is not an indication that anything is being accomplished and is certainly not an indication that anything is being done correctly. Such movements may not be doing anything or may be creating adverse effects. Adjustments should always be left to trained professionals.

The question of safety will likely arise when discussing adjustments. Knowing that the spine is a sensitive and essential part of the body, one would rightly wonder if manipulating it in this manner is safe. Clearly, the nature of chiropractic adjustments does introduce an element of risks just as any treatment protocol would.

Still, chiropractic care is recognized for being safe, medication free, and a non-invasive way of correcting problems caused by improper spinal alignment. Chiropractic care has a track record for being a safe method of treatment. With any treatment there is always a chance that there may be unforeseen consequences, but chiropractic care is known for being a method of treatment that is reliably without harmful effects the majority of the time.

PREGNANT WOMEN

A special case is that of pregnant women. Patients may wonder if chiropractic care can be administered when a woman is pregnant. The improved functioning of the body is advantageous for anyone. Because chiropractic care is individualized, the proper adjustments and amount of pressure are evaluated on a patient to patient basis and are therefore adjusted to any special needs of a patient, including pregnancy. Pregnant women who receive chiropractic treatments often report that the delivery goes more smoothly. There are even studies that indicate that chiropractic care can reduce the need for pain medications during the labor process and may even reduce the total time of the labor.

CHILDREN

This discussion has focused mainly on adult and how they experience and can benefit from chiropractic care, but do the same truths apply to children? Children are typically smaller and are still going through periods of rapid growth and development so can they benefit from chiropractic intervention? Indeed, the answer is once again an emphatic yes. Any individual who can benefit from proper alignment of the spine can benefit from some degree of chiropractic care.

Children may be subject to the same precipitating factors than can bring adults in for treatment. They may experience the same injuries or other causes of spinal misalignment and can likewise benefit from chiropractic adjustments.

Because the amount of force applied is already adjusted on a patient by patient basis, children are treated in the manner that is most suitable to them. The art of chiropractic care is individualized and transfers well to children. The application of pressure may be lessened, but the underlying principles are the same.

You may think of other special cases where you may think that the potential for chiropractic care may be questionable. You may wonder if everyone can truly benefit from chiropractic intervention. Again, the individualized nature of chiropractic treatment makes it all possible. By adjusting every treatment to the patient, chiropractic care remains as safe and as effective as possible. Anyone can benefit from correct spinal alignment so anyone who needs help in that area can benefit from chiropractic care.

4

BENEFITS OF CHIROPRACTIC CARE

There are many benefits that have been linked to chiropractic care. The most obvious are pain relief from acute or repetitive injuries, usually manifesting as pain in the back or as headaches, but the list does not end there.

Chiropractic care seeks to treat the cause of a problem and not just the symptoms. The benefit of this is that you really get to the root of the problem. By treating the condition that causes the symptoms instead of the symptoms themselves, chiropractors can eliminate all the symptoms that the condition produces. The benefits of such an approach are extensive. It would be best to begin an understanding of the results of chiropractic care with a basic exploration of the common problems that cause patients to seek out chiropractic care and how these problems may benefit from such care.

PAIN RELIEF

The topic of pain relief covers many areas of the body. It may begin with headaches and extend to a discussion of back pain, neck pain, and joint pain. Every case is unique so only a cursory explanation can be given, but this will help you to understand the general concept and principles at work.

Back pain, for instance, is more complicated than whether you have it or not. It may be located in different parts of the back. The pain may also be a dull feeling of discomfort or a sharp pain. You must also take into consideration if the pain is a constant presence or if it only appears when certain positions are assumed.

The severity of the pain is another factor. It may be a mild feeling of discomfort, or it may be agony. The pain may exist independently or it may coexist with numbness or tingling sensations.

Pain without tingling or numbness may be caused by spinal joint inflammation, muscle tears, poor posture, or improper lumbar curve. This is not an exhaustive list, but it allows you to see how what may seem to be a simple problem could be caused by a number of different conditions. Excess weight, especially around the midsection, can contribute to postural problems and may cause or worsen back pain.

Pain with tingling may be caused by disc bulges, disc degeneration, or herniated discs. These are only a few possible causes. Numbness or a tingling sensation is not natural in the body especially if said numbness is prolonged.

The treatment of back pain may include adjustments that seek to stretch the muscles and increase the range of motion of joints. These actions can diminish pain and any tension in the muscles while increasing a patient's mobility. The patient may also require additional therapy to strengthen the surrounding muscles, but chiropractic care alone can often reduce the patient's suffering and increase mobility.

Headaches are often thought of as a problem requiring some over the counter medication and then continuing with your day. They may, however, be caused by poor spinal alignment and can often be improved with the help of chiropractic acre. They, too, can have a myriad of causes and can range from mild headaches to migraines.

The use of chiropractic care to ameliorate symptoms is often effective for patients who suffer from headaches. In some cases, muscles at the base of the neck clench and tighten which can create tension in the neck and may be a contributing factor to headaches. Chiropractic care can intervene and often provide relief from the pain and tension associated with headaches.

Neck pain can be caused by poor posture, acute trauma, or degeneration. The lack of proper posture in the work place is an increasingly seen cause of neck problems and pain problems in general. Computer screens especially cause people to put their heads into awkward positions. A computer screen that is not properly placed forces an individual to tilt their head at an awkward angle and often forces them to do so for a prolonged period of time on a daily basis. Over time, this poor positioning is bound to create problems. The weight of the head is significant and can easily strain the muscles of the neck if the weight is not distributed equally as it is when an individual's posture is correct.

Chiropractic care can help to relieve pain and restore lost range of motion in the neck, allowing the patient to return to a natural position where the head is resting upon the neck and not leaning forward placing further undue strain on the neck. To maintain these results, the faulty ergonomics of the workplace will have to be fixed.

Shoulder pain is another injury centered on a joint that may very well benefit from chiropractic intervention. These injuries are made all the more important by the fact that people use their arms constantly in daily life. Shoulder pain may be cause by tendonitis, muscle tears, ligament tears, and any other of a number of conditions.

Injuries to the shoulder tend to be caused by a clearly identifiable traumatic experience although this is not always the case. Some shoulder injuries occur without a clear precipitating event.

Chiropractic treatments for shoulder injuries can prove helpful and are often used in conjunction with other healing modalities such as massage therapy. The joint and muscles must also undergo rehabilitation as the limited use experienced after the injury will necessitate it. To work towards healing the injury and then to return as much of the former joint mobility and strength as possible will probably require a combination of differing treatment modalities.

IMPROVED IMMUNE SYSTEM

Chiropractic care is also able to help your immune system function better. This is not surprising considering that the practice of chiropractic care assists the entire body to function better both as isolated parts and as a more cohesive whole. A body that is balanced is better equipped to defend itself against the immune system threats that many people face on a daily basis, and chiropractic treatment works toward that end.

A healthy immune system is said to be able to easily take care of the majority of the threats that it encounters on a daily basis. You have surely heard how proper nutrition, adequate sleep, and low stress levels help your body to stay healthy. Keeping your body balanced requires more than monitoring these outer influences. Your inner workings, including your spinal positioning, also have an effect.

A poorly positioned spinal column can interfere with the signals being sent from the brain to other parts of the body. It can even put pressure on nerves endings which, aside from causing pain, can inhibit the ability of your immune system to fight off invaders. The nervous system has dominion over all the systems of the body including the immune system. Proper spinal alignment allows for the proper functioning of everything else in the body, including the immune system.

Spinal misalignment can not only cause problems, but it can leave you more vulnerable to outside threats such as viruses. The proper alignment of the spine can restore order to the body, allow for an immune system that functions properly, and can help your body to repel invaders that it is naturally able to repel.

The systems of the body are not independent of each other. Poor functioning in one system affects all the other systems. It is one large integrated whole.

More than affecting one system, issues with the spine affect the communication that keeps the body running as it should. Slow or absent signals leave the body vulnerable and unable to defend itself from outside influences just as those affected signals can slow or prevent the body from healing already existing injuries.

You cannot have spinal misalignments and expect your immune system to be functioning properly. When your spinal positioning is impaired then your immune system follows.

Chiropractic care seeks to rectify these spinal misalignments and thereby restores the immune system to its natural state of functioning. As problems are corrected, the immune system becomes better able to take care of the body. The effects of chiropractic care are far reaching and even play a large part in the cold and fluseason.

OTHER BENEFITS

The other possible benefits of chiropractic care are endless. You are not just treating one isolated part of the body when you improve the alignment of the spine. You are allowing the entire system to function more efficiently.

This is another example of the system's integrated nature. When you correct alignment of nerve signals to one part of the body, you do not just work to ameliorate whatever condition brought that patient in for treatment in the first place. You also allow for clearer, faster signals to reach that entire region of the body.

The ability to treat isolated, discernable health conditions is a straightforward benefit of chiropractic treatment, but its effects also include a less describable improvement of the functioning of all bodily systems. Not all systems deteriorate to the point where the need for improvement is obvious. Some systems have a less discernible downward slide that may not even be noticed until their full potential is once again restored and realized.

Many benefits of chiropractic care have been observed both by science and by anecdotal evidence from patients themselves. It is true that one must take into account the possibility of a placebo effect wherein patients simply convince themselves that they are experiencing an improvement in their symptoms regardless of the efficacy of a treatment protocol, but the consistent nature of positive feedback and the research that has supported these claims is difficult to ignore. The benefits of chiropractic care for patients are very real.

You may view the ability to treat back problems, neck problems, and problems with the spine without having to resort to surgery as a major benefit of chiropractic services. Chiropractic care may not allow patients to avoid surgery in all cases, but it has allowed many to forego this invasive maneuver.

The word invasive is not used in this case to mean that it is entirely detrimental. Rather, surgery can do a lot of good when necessary. It is only meant that surgery by its very nature is an invasive procedure. This description separates it from chiropractic care which is non-invasive and only seeks to rearrange what is already present in the body. It works with the body in its natural form as opposed to forcibly entering the body to make alterations.

It has also been noted that the lungs may be freed up and breathing may be improved through the utilization of chiropractic services. This is easily understood as chiropractic adjustments may restore the body to its correct posture which maximizes the space available for lungs to expand during each breath. A person who is hunched over may be physically restricting breathing through posture so a reversal of this postural abnormality would restore breathing capacity. Because respiratory functioning is such an important part of the overall functioning of the body, this restoration of breathing capacity is no small accomplishment.

It has been noted that chiropractic care has managed to improve conditions such as the common cold, allergies, and asthma in some patients. After gaining a working knowledge of how the body works and how chiropractic care improves the state of the body as a complete entity, this is not surprising. This ability to improve numerous health afflictions is in addition to the way that this treatment has been known to aid of the nervous system in its functioning as well as assisting the functioning of the heart and the coronary arteries. The effects of chiropractic care seem to go well into every system of the body in practice as well as in theory.

Some patients also experience a better feeling of overall health. This may included lessened anxiety, depression, and tension. By allowing some patients to relax and improve their mood state, the effects of chiropractic treatment extend further into the promotion of an overall sense of well being. Aside from the feeling of relief that surely accompanies a reduction in pain and physical problems, these results can often be found when chiropractic care is used solely as a preventativemeasure.

Finally, chiropractic care has been known to increase a patient's energy level and, of course, improve the patient's ability to heal. With all the benefits that chiropractic care can provide, it is no wonder that this alternative method of healing continues to grow in popularity.

5

THE PHILOSOPHY OF CHIROPRACTIC CARE

Chiropractic care is sometimes thought of as an alternative method of dealing with health problems. The traditional methods may include the aforementioned options of medications and surgery. Both are, arguably, invasive and depend upon forces from outside of the patient's body to complete the healing process.

Ideally, the body should be able to heal itself. It has a remarkable capacity for regeneration. This assumes that the body's basic needs are met and that the body is properly maintained. You would not expect a weakened body to be able to perform as well in physical activities as a healthy body so too should you not expect a body that has been weakened by spinal misalignment to be able to perform as well as a healthy body.

While physical activity may be an outward and easily recognized demonstration of inner weakness, the immune system also reflects the health of the body as a whole. If the body is not balanced and maintained then the immune system cannot work at peak efficiency. If a body were out of balance in some other way then this weakening may be more obvious to the casual observer.

If a person were malnourished, for example, you would have no problem linking all the resulting functional deficiencies and internal problems to the malnutrition. So, too, spinal misalignment pervades the many systems, cells, and processes of the body just as proper nutrition does. You would not expect an individual's body to be as able to fight off infection if they were malnourished. Similarly, a body weakened by poor spinal alignment cannot express its full immune system potential either.

Chiropractic care has as its goal the restoration of the natural ability of the body to heal. It wishes to avoid, whenever possible, going to outside sources to aid in the healing process. One might argue that chiropractic care itself is an outside influence, and this is true to an extent. It is an outside influence, but it only works with the tools already present in the human body.

Instead of introducing something new or removing something from the body, chiropractic care hopes to adjust the body and retrain it to once again embrace its natural state. In its natural state the human body has the ability to take over in the healing process and to take care of any problems in a natural way.

HOW IT DIFFERS FROM TRADITIONAL MEDICINE

Traditional medicine seeks to treat the body using resources from outside of the body. The belief is that something is wrong with the body and must be fixed. It is sometimes believed that only those trained professionals in the medical field have the ability to fix a basically "broken" body by introducing some outside influence into the system.

This may be accomplished through the influence of medications or through surgical procedures.

For example, pain may be treated with medications, and muscle injuries may be treated through various surgical procedures. In both instances, foreign influences are used to attempt to fix problems. These techniques, while they have the best of intentions, may be detrimental to the body.

Medications are outside influences on the body. They may have side effects that are often difficult to predict. These adverse effects occur because the medication seeks to provide an influence that the body cannot produce or is currently unable to produce on its own.

Medications have different reactions when they are introduced into different individuals. There is not always one medication that improves a condition for every patient. Instead, there are several choices of medications that must be gone through in a process of trial and error.

Medications meant to help have the potential to harm because their exact effects in a patient's body are unknown. Surely, there has to be a better method than attempting to give patients medication with unknown effects. Medications cannot be the best substitutes for natural bodily chemicals in all cases.

It would be preferable if there were no need for substitutes at all. If the body were restored to a state of proper functioning then it may be able to produce the correct form of the chemical on its own without having to rely on a synthetic that may attempt to be a substitute but that may not be as effective or effective at all.

This may not always point to chiropractic care, but the philosophy extends beyond one particular method of healing. It is an ideology wherein the simplest, most natural techniques of healing are preferred over invasive techniques that can do harm even as they attempt to promote healing.

If something you were eating was making you sick then you would stop eating it. If something you did was causing you pain then you could stop doing it. You would not want to continue doing something that was harming you just because you could take a pill that would make you numb to its unpleasant effects.

In the case of pills for pain, you would still be doing damage to your system even if you could not feel it. You have not fixed the problem of spinal misalignment. You would only be hiding from it until it once again became impossible to ignore. In such cases, taking pills hides the problem from your sight instead of dealing with it.

Likewise, surgery is invasive. This is not to say that surgery is unnecessary or not a valuable medical tool. In many cases surgery has proven to be helpful for patients with certain conditions. However, in cases where surgery can be avoided, it surely would be a better option to allow the body to heal itself as opposed to forcibly entering the body to make the necessary adjustments.

In cases where something adjustable such as spinal misalignment is causing the problem, the spine may be adjusted to affect the appropriate repairs. The healing could begin and end within the body. If you were to use surgery in a case where spinal misalignment was the source of or a contributing factor to the problem then you may be able to repair the immediate problems but not the circumstances that caused it.

You would be, in essence, buying time. The condition could surely return because the factors that caused it have not been corrected. You would have fixed a symptom of the problem and not the problem itself.

Chiropractic care attempts to, in as unobtrusive a way as possible, help the patient's body to help itself. It views the body as already complete and often able to affect its own repairs if only allowed to do so.

As previously explained, the spinal column is the route through which signals are sent from the brain to the rest of the body. Spinal misalignment can result in obstructed pathways which can then cause health problems and a decreased ability to heal from those problems.

Chiropractic care seeks to correct the effects of daily life, such as poor posture so that the patient's body may be returned to a more natural state. Once the body is returned to a more natural state then it is more able to complete repairs on its own.

This method of healing does not truly add or remove anything to or from the body. Rather, it uses the potential already within the body, which may be impeded by spinal misalignment, and seeks to reawaken this dormant potential.

This difference in the philosophy of healing is the most noteworthy aspect of this separation between ideas of healing. Traditional medicine sees the body as having something wrong with it that must be corrected.

Someone, presumably a doctor or a surgeon, must go into the body in some manner and correct whatever is wrong. This may be through surgery or through the use of prescription medications. This approach can be problematic because it seeks, in many cases, to remove the problem.

While removing the problem can be helpful and even life saving in some situations, it can easily overlook the issues that causes the health problem in the first place. It can overlook the basic cause and effect chain of events that is occurring within the body. If this chain of causation is overlooked and the resulting medical condition is corrected then the circumstance which caused it may remain. This circumstance may create the same problem again.

It is similar to removing a quantity of fat from a person's body without changing their nutritional intake or their exercise habits. Once the operation is completed then the deposits of fat will be replaced because the circumstances that initially caused them, the poor diet or lack of exercise, are still present. You have not dealt with the cause of the condition. You have only attempted to fix one of the symptoms. This does not benefit the patient in the long term.

Similarly, you can take a pill for cholesterol or high blood pressure, but if it is an individual's nutritional intake that is causing or contributing to the problem then you have not dealt with the real cause of the problem. You are attempting to use an artificial means to heal the body when, given the right circumstances, the body could possibly heal itself.

Chiropractic care seeks to give the body that chance to heal itself. With spinal manipulation, it attempts to create the proper circumstances for the body to begin this process of self-healing. Nothing is really introduced into the body, and nothing is taken away. Instead, the body is brought back into
58

its natural balance and then allowed to repair and heal itself as it would naturally because this is the natural way for the body to heal.

It may seem simpler to circumvent this process and attempt to treat the problem with a pill, but it does not benefit the patient in the long run.

You can take medications to avoid feeling the pain in your back, but the problem is still there. You have only masked it. There is a problem with masking it.

If your problem has progressed to the point where it is causing you pain then it may continue to progress, and it may once again become a problem you cannot ignore. This time it will be worse because you did not correct the cause when the symptoms first began to manifest to alert you that something was wrong.

It would seem that anyone would agree that the best course of action would be to allow the body to perform its own healing in its own way and in its own time. The body has an innate wisdom all its own. It is a remarkable construct that has a keen awareness for what it does and does not need. Given the right circumstances, self-healing is often a distinct possibility. Chiropractic care provides those right circumstances.

This is not a dismissal of traditional medical practices but a call for re- examination of them. Are they still the best methods that medical professionals have at their disposal? Could these changes in the human body be completed in another manner? Is it time for a re-evaluation of society's very notion of the healing process?

A shift from the idea of something being wrong with the body and a need for outside forces to fix it could become an idea of a body that is out of balance that needs to have its balance restored. Once restored to a more natural balanced state then the body could be left to its own innate, intuitive healing ability.

6

WHY CHIROPRACTIC CARE MIGHT
BE RIGHT FOR YOU

It may be beneficial to end with a review of the basics of chiropractic care. Chiropractic care seeks to help your body to heal itself. This perspective has been present since the beginning of recorded history. It has evolved into a science that requires thorough training for all those who wish to be licensed to practice.

Chiropractic science is based on the fact that the spine is a conduit for messages to travel to and from the brain. This is the vehicle through which the brain affects the body and through which signals are relayed back to the brain. The state of the spine can affect the entire body's ability to function.

In chiropractic care, a qualified professional first evaluates a patient and that patient's spinal alignment to see if chiropractic care is a viable method of treatment for the issues at hand. If other methods of healing might be beneficial in conjunction with chiropractic treatment then those too can be employed to help the patient.

A chiropractor applies pressure to retrain the spine to assume its proper alignment. This is the common image of this healing modality, and it is heart of the physical practice of chiropractic care.

Because chiropractic care seeks to fix the circumstances that created the problems in the first place, it seeks out a lasting solution. A pill may make you feel better, but it may not fix the underlying issue. It is only by rectifying the underlying issue that a patient finds true lasting relief. This is the philosophy that underlies the practice of chiropractic treatment.

This may seem to be an alternative approach for a society that prefers instant cures, but true healing must deal with the underlying issues. True healing takes time.

Chiropractic care is not about avoiding other avenues of healing. It is about finding the most effective, natural, and least intrusive method for a patient to heal.

Chiropractic care helps your body to heal itself the natural way. You can ignore the pain or you can take a pill to make it go away, but in many cases this only avoids the matter at hand. These actions or a state of inaction will not necessarily heal the problem and may even allow your condition to get worse.

Would you want to have surgery when your body may be able to heal itself with a little help? Would you want to take a pill knowing that the problem may still be there even if you no longer feel it? Do you want a body that has the ability to heal itself?

Chiropractic care is all about natural healing. It is meant to restore the natural order that your body needs to function at its best. Because the nature of chiropractic care leads it to restore order to a system that impacts so much of your health, you may not just heal the problems that you have. You might avoid future problems and improve your overall health, and you can do it in a natural way. These are the benefits of chiropractic care.

9 786069 836958

Printed by Libri Plureos GmbH in Hamburg, Germany